Vabitha Shetty
Amitha Hegde

Silver Diamine Fluoride in Pediatric Dentistry

Shivani Daga
Vabitha Shetty
Amitha Hegde

Silver Diamine Fluoride in Pediatric Dentistry

the knight in shining armour

LAP LAMBERT Academic Publishing

Imprint
Any brand names and product names mentioned in this book are subject to trademark, brand or patent protection and are trademarks or registered trademarks of their respective holders. The use of brand names, product names, common names, trade names, product descriptions etc. even without a particular marking in this work is in no way to be construed to mean that such names may be regarded as unrestricted in respect of trademark and brand protection legislation and could thus be used by anyone.

Cover image: www.ingimage.com

Publisher:
LAP LAMBERT Academic Publishing
is a trademark of
International Book Market Service Ltd., member of OmniScriptum Publishing Group
17 Meldrum Street, Beau Bassin 71504, Mauritius

ISBN: 978-620-0-78457-5

Copyright © Shivani Daga, Vabitha Shetty, Amitha Hegde
Copyright © 2020 International Book Market Service Ltd., member of OmniScriptum Publishing Group

CONTENTS

1	INTRODUCTION	3-7
2	MECHANISM OF ACTION	8-11
3	CLINICAL APPLICATIONS	12-16
4	DISADVANTAGES	17-21

5	STUDIES DONE ON SDF	22-27
6	AAPD GUIDELINES	28-32
7	CONCLUSION	33-34
8	BIBLIOGRAPHY	35-43

1. INTRODUCTION

Dental caries is a multifactorial bacterial driven disease which results in demineralization of the tooth structure over a period of time posing health problems to mankind. Data from caries epidemiological surveys reflects that in both developed and developing countries dental caries is a significant disease present in childhood. It is still a major problem in many societies and in children belonging to disadvantaged communities. The prevalence of caries in children is high in families with low income, lower education level of parents, poor parental dental attitude.

The child's ability to perform their routine activities, dietary patterns and sleep is greatly affected if caries left untreated, thereby affecting their oral and general well-being. [1]

The prevailing methods adopted in industrialized countries for the prevention and treatment of dental caries are not affordable in developing countries where there are inadequate financial resources, dental manpower and facilities.

Further, treating dental caries in young children can be very cumbersome as the child has limited coping abilities and the poor cooperation makes it very challenging for the dentist to remove all the caries and provide a restoration.[2]

It was proposed that rather than leaving caries untreated in children of disadvantaged communities, arresting caries treatment is an alternative treatment protocol without immediate restorative intervention.[3] The use of topical fluorides may be a useful measure to arrest caries lesions because fluorides used in various forms have proven to be effective in dental caries prevention. [4]

Fluoride exerts its caries-protective properties in several ways. The primary anti-caries effect is a topical effect on erupted teeth.[5] Fluoride concentrated in plaque and saliva can inhibit demineralization of dental hard tissue.[6] Fluoride taken up along with calcium and phosphate by demineralized dental hard tissue forms a crystalline structure (demineralization) that is more resistant to the challenges of bacterial acid.[7] Fluoride has also been shown to inhibit the process by which cariogenic bacteria metabolize carbohydrates to produce acids, and thus affect the bacterial production of adhesive polysaccharides.[7]

Silver diamine fluoride is an inexpensive topical fluoride(SDF) which has been shown to halt the carious process and also prevents the occurrence of newer carious lesions. It is a colourless aqueous solution that contains silver and fluoride ions which provides antimicrobial and remineralizing properties. It is used in dentistry to promote remineralisation of tooth mineral hydroxyapatite that is under constant acid challenge in the oral cavity.

SDF has been used to deal with high caries prevalence by arresting or slowing down the rate of caries progression It has been successfully used for arresting caries in primary teeth. It is also used in the management of dental caries in young children , to arrest root caries , to prevent pit and fissure caries , to prevent secondary caries , to desensitize sensitive teeth , to treat infected root canals and to prevent the fracture of endodontically treated teeth. [2]

Several clinical studies and extensive research work in the 21st century established SDF as a safe and effective anti caries agent. This evoked a revival of interest in this potential fluoride agent. [2]

In August 2014, the Food and Drug Administration cleared the first SDF product which was readily available in market. Its beneficial properties as an effective caries control agent appears to meet both the world health organization millennium goals and the US Institute of Medicine's criteria for 21st century medical care. [8]

BACKGROUND

The first medicinal use for silver appears to have been around 1000 BC for the storing of potable water. Uses of silver compounds in medicine revolve around the application of silver nitrate, silver foil, and silver sutures for the prevention of ocular and surgical infections. Naegeli et al demonstrated that silver can kill spirogyra, and found that various forms of silver have different effects, with silver nitrate being a very effective antimicrobial agent.[9]

In dentistry, Since the 1840s silver compounds have been used widely because of its antimicrobial and anti-caries properties. Silver nitrate and Howe's solution were actively used for caries management during this period.[10] However, when antibiotics came to the market, it was proved superior to silver compounds in their efficacy to combat infections and in the ease of manufacture.[11] This led to a decline in the research and clinical interest in silver compounds. Gradually there was antibacterial resistance seen with some antibiotics and in the 1970s there was a reappearance of the interest in silver compounds.[12]

The silver and fluoride was combined presuming that it would have a substantial beneficial effect as an anti caries agent and will also aid in remineralization. Its use was initiated in Japan in the late 1960s and 1970s and was supported by central
pharmaceutical council of the ministry of health and welfare. Along with its clinical implication to arrest caries, it blackened the carious lesions thereby limiting its use.[13]

A clinician in Mexico had reported that a 2-year-old child who had caries in the incisors associated with a nursing bottle had the caries arrested and hardened after the use of sodium fluoride (NaF) and silver nitrate solution (Aron, 1995).SDF in various concentrations has been used in community dental health projects in Argentina, Brazil and Spain; and further community projects were planned for sub-Saharan Africa and for several other African countries.[3]

Although an article in an American journal mentioned that there were clinicians in Southern California who used SDF to arrest caries and to harden the demineralised dentine of young children with early childhood caries.[14] The school dental service in Western Australia used 40% silver fluoride (AgF) as the standard treatment for deep caries lesions in primary teeth. Beneficial results were reported by Craig et al (1981) when using AgF followed by SnF2 solution to arrest caries in primary molars in very young children who were difficult to manage.[15]

The use of SDF was quite scarce during this period and not much literature is available in English during this period.

Over the last 40 years, numerous preliminary in vitro and in vivo trials examined the potential efficacy of silver-fluoride regimens in caries prevention.

In vitro studies suggested that silver fluoride regimens inhibit S. mutans growth, metabolic activity of dental plaque and caries lesion depth progression (Klein *et al.*, no date). Similarly, in vivo studies in primary teeth indicated that silver-fluoride application inhibit the lateral spread of caries, using SDF.[13] occlusal and proximal caries by silver diamine and stannous fluoride and 95% of caries progress using SDF + SnF2.[17] In vivo studies in permanent teeth indicated that silver fluoride arrests proximal caries progression using Silver nitrate (AgNO3) and also the initiation of caries lesion.[18]

At the beginning of the 21st century, several studies were carried out in China and its use was popularised again when SDF solution was applied to primary teeth of school children.

Chu et al. carried out a study on the use of SDF in arresting carious lesions in 370 Chinese pre-school children aged three to five years old. They compared groups of children receiving SDF treatment, sodium fluoride varnish and a control. The children were followed up for 30 months receiving an intervention every three months.

Children in the SDF groups had a mean of 2.8 arrested lesions compared with a mean of 1.5 in the varnish group. They were able to conclude that the application of an SDF solution was more effective in arresting dentine caries in primary teeth compared with sodium fluoride varnish.[19]

Similar results were echoed in a study by Lo et al. which followed 375 Chinese pre-school children over an 18-month period comparing groups of children receiving treatment with SDF, NaF varnish and a control. They found a mean of 0.4 new carious lesions in the SDF treated group compared with 1.2 in the control. They also found similar results in arresting active carious lesions with a mean of 2.8 arrested lesions in the SDF group compared to 1.5 in the NaF varnish group.[20]

Therefore, these studies led to significant gain of interest in use of SDF for prevention and treatment of caries worldwide based on its ability to reduce instances of pain, ease of use, affordability, non-invasive property and minimum chair side time for application.

2. MECHANISM OF ACTION

The mechanism of the cariostatic action of SDF can be explained by the reaction products between SDF and mineral component of the tooth. Selvig et al showed that the fluoride treatment increased the resistance of the peri- and inter-tubular dentin to acid decalcification and as a result, retarded the penetration of acid into deeper layers of the dentin. [21] It has been reported that SDF ($Ag(NH_3)_2F$) when applied on tooth surface reacts with the tooth mineral hydroxyapatite (HA)($Ca_{10}(PO_4)_6(OH)_2$) to release calcium fluoride (CaF_2) and silver phosphate (Ag_3PO_4), which are responsible for the prevention and hardening of dental caries. Hydroxyapatite and fluoroapatite form on the exposed organic matrix, along with the presence of silver chloride and metallic silver.

A simplified chemical reaction was suggested as shown below. [20,13]

$$Ca_{10}(PO_4)_6(OH)_2 + Ag(NH_3)_2 \rightarrow CaF_2 + Ag_3PO_4 + NH_4OH$$
$$CaF_2 \rightarrow Ca^{++} + 2F^-$$
$$Ca_{10}(PO_4)_6(OH)_2 + 2F^- \rightarrow Ca_{10}(PO_4)_6F_2 + 2OH^-$$

The Ag_3PO_4 that precipitates on the tooth surface is insoluble and forms the squamous layer of conjugate from precipitation of silver-protein complex, increasing resistance to acid dissolution and enzymatic digestion.

The CaF_2 formed provides a reservoir of fluoride for the formation of fluorapatite ($Ca_{10}(PO_4)_6F_2$). Fluorapatite is stable and resists decalcification by acid and chelating agent, which is more resistant to acid attack than HA ($Ca_{10}(PO_4)_6(OH)_2$).[22] The treated lesion increases in mineral density and hardness while the lesion depth decreases, in addition, it is known that fluoride ions promote calcification, and also restores lattice imperfection. [23] and improves the crystallinity of HA.[24]

Meanwhile, silver diamine fluoride specifically inhibits the proteins that break down the exposed dentin organic matrix: matrix metalloproteinase, cathepsins; and bacterial collagenases. Its antibacterial properties arise from inhibition of the enzyme activities and dextran-induced agglutination of cariogenic strains of *Streptococcus mutans*.[25] It-might be attributing to reaction of Ag and organic component of dentin.[26] Yanagida *et al*. showed that dentin protein treated with Ag(NH3)2F had increased resistance to collagenase and trypsin.[27] Silver ions act directly against bacteria in lesions by breaking membranes, denaturing proteins, and inhibiting DNA replication. Ionic silver deactivates nearly any macromolecule.

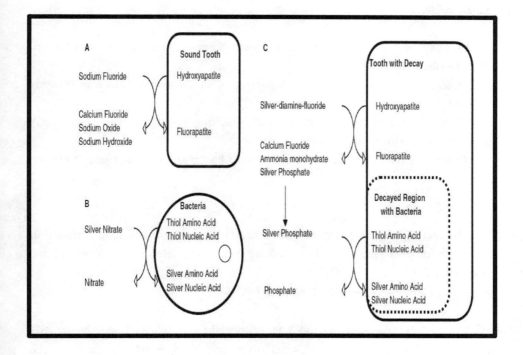

Diagrams representing effects of fluoride, silver nitrate, and silver diamine fluoride on teeth and bacteria. (Rosenblatt, Stamford and Niederman, 2009)[9]

There is various mechanism of actions depicted in the schematic diagram by which SDF reacts with:

(A) In sound teeth, fluoride reacts with hydroxyapatite to form fluorapatite. Fluorapatite is less acid-soluble than hydroxyapatite, inhibiting the decay process.

(B) In bacteria, silver reacts with thiol groups of amino and nucleic acids. Silver amino and nucleic acids are unable to carry out metabolic and reproductive functions, leading to bacterial killing.

(C) In teeth with decay, silver diamine fluoride reacts with hydroxyapatite to form fluorapatite, and the by-product silver phosphate. Silver phosphate subsequently reacts with bacterial amino and nucleic acid thiol groups to form silver amino and nucleic acids.

Multiple modes of action have been proposed for silver. (Lansdown, 2002)(Oerther, 2007) [28,29]

Studies have indicated that silver interacts with sulfhydryl groups of proteins and with
DNA, altering hydrogen bonding and inhibiting respiratory processes, DNA unwinding, cell-wall synthesis, and cell division.[30,31]

At the macro level, these interactions effect bacterial killing and inhibit biofilm formation (Oerther, 2007).[29]

The central mechanism for these diverse effects is proposed to be the interaction of silver with thiol groups by the following mechanism (Rosenblatt, Stamford and Niederman, 2009)[9]:

$$A/N - SH + AgX \rightarrow A/N\text{-}S\text{-}AgX + HX$$

where A/N represents amino (A) or nucleic (N) acids (respectively), SH represents a thiol group, Ag represents silver, and X represents an anion (in the current example, diamine fluoride).

This interaction indicates how silver diamine fluoride, when applied to caries lesions, might interact with bacteria and mediate caries arrest through bacterial killing and inhibit caries progress through the inhibition of biofilm formation.

Artificial lesions treated with silver diamine fluoride are resistant to biofilm formation and further cavity formation, presumably due to remnant ionic silver.[32,33] More silver and fluoride is deposited in demineralized than non-demineralized dentin; correspondingly, treated demineralized dentin is more resistant to caries bacteria than treated sound dentin.[34]

When bacteria killed by silver ions are added to living bacteria, the silver is reactivated, so that effectively the dead bacteria kill the living bacteria in a "zombie effect." This reservoir effect helps explain why silver deposited on bacteria and dentin proteins within a cavity has sustained antimicrobial effects.[35]

Suzuki *et al.* studied the mechanism of antiplaque action of diamine silver fluoride (Ag(NH3)2F). This agent showed excellent antibacterial action against cariogenic strains of *S. mutans* (minimal inhibitory concentration, 0.12 μmole/ml), and completely inhibited the dextran induced agglutination of *S. mutans* at 0.59 μmole/ml and sucrase activities of *S. mutans* at 0.2 μmole/ml. These effects were found to be the result of the action of silver ion. These results indicate that silver ion may inhibit the colonization of *S. mutans* on enamel surface and offer a possible explanation for the antiplaque action of the agent.[25]

Silver diamine fluoride outperforms other anti-caries medicaments in killing cariogenic bacteria in dentinal tubules for two reasons:

1. Silver and fluoride ions penetrate ~25 microns into enamel,16 and 50-200 microns into dentin. Fluoride promotes remineralisation, and silver is available for antimicrobial action Silver diamine fluoride arrested lesions are 150 microns thick.[8]

2. The binding of glucan to HA was inhibited by the treatment of HA with fluoride solution, but was slightly promoted by that with silver solution.[2]

Understanding the mechanism of action of SDF will be helpful in determining its clinical application.

3. CLINICAL APPLICATIONS

To deal with the high caries prevalence and management problem of young children with a minimal invasion approach.

First proposal to use this approach was made by Yamaga *et al.* in Japan. The most common approach to deal with dental caries is to use rotary dental handpiece, spoon excavators to remove the infected dentin.[27] A difficulty for the dental practitioner especially dealing with young children, is the use of conventional rotary instrument, often thought of as a "drill" or pressure from spoon excavator are often cited as triggering patient fear and anxiety. As silver diamine fluoride has an ability to arrest caries, it can be considered as a useful approach to deal with such young patient. Once the carious process is slowed down or arrested, caries removal can be done at later date when child's ability to rationalize fear is increased with age.

In pre-school children, many primary teeth are attacked by caries, and a very large number of the children have "early childhood caries" which takes an acute course. However, the treatment of such carious deciduous teeth involves many difficulties, so a majority of the patients are left untreated at present.[2]

Primary teeth not only play an important role in the normal eruption and growth of the permanent teeth, but also are essential for the growth of the jaw bone which is the growth and development of the face.

From such a point of view, it may be reasonable to sacrifice the aesthetic factor to a certain extent, if the progress of dental caries can be arrested by the application of the solution. Previous approach to rampant caries was to remove possible carious dentin and use zinc oxide eugenol as temporary restoration. Unfortunately, the pattern of caries is so irregular that zinc oxide eugenol cannot be retained in all the cavitated surfaces. SDF can provide a better alternative for the same.

As a topical fluoride agent for prevention of caries.

Silver diamine fluoride can also be used as a topical fluoride agent. As it has the property to reduce *S. mutans* count, it can also prevent initiation of caries and remineralize incipient carious lesions. Two *in vitro* studies have shown contradictory results:

Initially Suzuki *et al.* evaluated that fluoride concentration of the enamel treated with SDF was similar to those of sodium fluoride and stannous fluoride. The percent ratio of the concentration of retained fluoride to that of uptake fluoride was highest when enamel was treated with SDF. On the other hand, Delbem *et al.* found that fluoridated varnish was more effective to reduce both the enamel surface demineralization and caries lesion depth than SDF solution. [22]

In another study by Najmeh et al, enamel blocks treated with SDF and fluoride varnish showed higher quantitative resistance to demineralization compared to the control group. Even though this difference was not statistically significant, it can be substantial

in clinical use.[36] In a study by Chu *et al.*, it was shown that SDF is more effective on dentinal carious lesions. The reason is that dentinal tissue has a higher content of protein, carbonate, and phosphate available to react with silver. In contrast, these compounds are scarce in enamel tissue. More studies are required to conclude the fluoride uptake by enamel from SDF.[37]

To prevent secondary caries

True adhesion has been the "holy grail" of dental restorative materials for many decades. Since most restorative materials used in general dentistry today truly adhere to the tooth structure or completely insoluble in oral fluids; saliva, bacteria and food debris penetrate through the space between the cavity walls and the restorative materials.[38] Hence, the cavity wall may always be in danger of recurrent caries.

To inhibit recurrent caries, therefore, resistance of cavity wall to caries must be enhanced. Shimizu and Kawagoe (1976) found no recurrent caries on amalgam restorations on primary teeth pre-treated with SDF after 26 months.[39]

To prevent pit and fissure caries

Pits and fissures are more susceptible to dental caries than the smooth surface for Morphological reasons. It is also difficult to clean pits and fissures with a toothbrush. While it is difficult to discover incipient lesion at pits and fissures, the topical fluoride

Application is revealed far less effective for the prevention of the pit and fissure caries than that of the smooth surface.

According to Sato *et al* due to its antibacterial and caries preventive property, SDF can be effective for the prevention of pits and fissures caries of the first molar teeth. [40]

Nishino and Massler (1977) in their study mentioned that caries score of Ag(NH3)2F treated teeth was significantly lower than the fissures treated with SnF2 8% or Ag(NO)3. [41]

The application should be recorded as a precaution because of greyish-black and black stain at the pit and fissure by SDF may be mistaken for incipient caries.

In community dental health programs

SDF can be used to tackle the caries problem in community dental health programs in developing countries. The main advantages as pointed out by Bedi and Infirri (1999) are as follows [3]

• Control of pain and infection. SDF is effective in arresting caries progression that if left untreated will cause pain and infection Affordable cost.

• The cost of SDF treatment is low and should be affordable in most communities simplicity of treatment.

• The procedures are simple. This allows non dental professionals including primary health care workers to be easily trained to apply SDF to children minimal support required.

• The treatment does not require expensive equipment or support infrastructure such as piped water and electricity.

• Non-invasive procedure, the treatment is non-invasive and thus the risk of spreading infection is very low.

As an agent for atraumatic restorative technique

Quock *et al*. proposed hypothesis regarding drill less feeling. A drill-less filling will involve the utilization of SDF (38%) to arrest and prevent dental caries, followed by restoration with a bonded filling material to achieve adequate seal at the lesion margins. Hence, more research is required to evaluate the hypothesis. [42]

Santos et al. examined whether, for underprivileged school children with cavities, treatment with 30% SDF gives better results than intermediate restorative technique (IRT) (Glass ionomer cement [GIC]) for carries arrest. [43]

After 1 year, The SDF technique showed better results than intermediate restorative technique(IRT) for arresting cavities in deciduous teeth, indicating that its use for underprivileged communities may justify a paradigm shift in pediatric dentistry.

To arrest root caries
Epidemiological studies have shown that the incidence of root caries increases with age,(Griffin et al., 2004) [44] and the prevalence of root caries in elders are high. [45,46]

Two different studies by Tan et al. (2010) and Zhang et al. (2013) mentioned that due to its high ability to arrest dental caries, annual application of SDF is quite effective in arresting the caries on root surfaces. [47,48]

To desensitize sensitive teeth
As suggested by Gottlieb, there is a common factor between the mechanism of desensitizing hypersensitive dentin and arresting dental caries and it may be possible to evaluate the caries-arresting effect of an agent in terms of the desensitizing action. As SDF has an ability to occlude the dentinal tubule it can give promising results in patients with dentinal hypersensitivity. [2]

There are a number of constituents in the diamine silver fluoride / potassium iodide preparations that could have contributed to the significant reduction in dentine hypersensitivity observed in this study. Silver ions can precipitate proteins in the dentinal tubules and have a long history of use as a dentine desensitizing agent. Fluoride ions can react with free calcium ions to form deposits of calcium fluoride that can block dentinal tubules. Also, the formation of silver iodide from the reaction between diamine silver fluoride and potassium iodide when used in combination have been sufficient to contribute further to a reduction in dentine tubule patency. [15]

Hatsuyama et al. Murase et al. and Kimura et al have shown that (Ag(NH3)2F) was the most effective against erosion and abrasion followed hypersensitive dentin to mechanical, cold, and heat sensation. It was also suggested that 4 times repeated application was the most appropriate application protocol. [2]

Apart from the above-mentioned clinical implications, SDF can also be used for below-mentioned situation. Further research is required to accept it for the particular usage.

As an Indirect pulp capping agent.

As described by Yamaga et al. [17] if SDF is applied in the presence of softened dentin, it will arrest the subsequent progress of dental caries. This may be considered to indicate that, in case a small amount of softened dentin remains after preparation of cavities or abutment teeth, or when the softened dentin cannot be completely removed for a risk of exposing the pulp, the application of SDF renders the residual softened dentin harmless.

In animal experiment SDF exerted no serious effect histologically on the pulp by application to the medium deep cavity, and in application to human deciduous teeth with moderate dentin caries the agent exerted no clinical symptoms. Chu and Lo in their review article also proposed to use SDF as caries arresting agent in atraumatic restorative technique and as an indirect pulp capping (IPC) agents. Until date, no reported study is found in this direction in primary teeth. [14]

Gupta et al. in their *in vitro* study found highest zone of bacterial inhibition was found with SDF. [49] *In vivo* part of the same study done by Sinha et al. and it was mentioned that SDF has remineralizing, re-hardening and antimicrobial efficacy and hence can act as effective indirect pulp capping materials. [50]

4. DISADVANTAGES

The inherent drawback of using SDF to arrest caries is that the lesions will be stained black as shown in the figure below. Therefore, some children and their parents may not be pleased with the aesthetics of this treatment outcome.

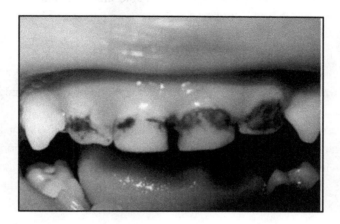

Black stain on SDF-treated lesions was commonly found, particularly in the groups with a higher SDF concentration and more frequent application. The clinical success of SDF application in arresting active caries lesion may be positively correlated with the presence of a protective layer appearing as a black stain over the lesion.

In the same study, Despite the black stains, the proportion of parents who were satisfied with their children's dental appearance at the 30-months follow-up was higher than that at baseline, possible because parents' satisfaction is complex and multidimensional. [19]

If the risk versus benefit is to be evaluated rather than leaving the child without any treatment of dental caries which will lead to discomfort, aesthetic concerns can be sacrificed and importance of caries control process can be explained to the parent.

In Hong Kong, there is no public or subsidized dental service for preschool children; thus, access to conventional restorative care is low. Health care system and cultural beliefs may have an impact on parents' perception toward SDF treatment.

Other aspects, such as tooth alignment and dental caries status of their children, may influence their satisfaction. [51]

Social class significantly contributed to parental satisfaction, Parents with lower socioeconomic status were more likely to be satisfied with the treatment outcome; this implies that SDF would be more acceptable among parents in disadvantaged communities in which early childhood caries is more prevalent. [52]

It has been suggested that when carious dentin was treated with SDF, silver phosphate was formed, and this was insoluble. Silver phosphate is yellow when it is first formed, but readily turns black under sunlight or the influence of reducing agents.

To overcome this limitation Knight et al. proposed to used Potassium iodide after application of SDF to the tooth structure remaining free silver ions in solution will react with Potassium Iodide to precipitate creamy white silver iodide crystals. Hence, free silver ions no longer available to react with sulfur and other reagents in the mouth to form black precipitates into the teeth. [15]

This is an off-label use; potassium iodide is approved as an over the counter drug to facilitate mucus release to breathe more easily with chronic lung problems, and to protect the thyroid from radioactive iodine in radiation emergencies. In clinical experience, SSKI helps but does not dramatically effect stain; arrested lesions normally darken. [8]

Most stain remains at the dentin-enamel or cementum-enamel junction. However, SSKI maintains resistance to biofilm formation or activity in laboratory studies. [33] Also, SSKI maintained caries arrest efficacy in the early results of an ongoing clinical trial. [53]

SSKI is contraindicated in pregnant women and during the first six months of breastfeeding due to concern of overloading the developing thyroid with iodide; thyroid specialists suggested a pregnancy test prior to use in women of childbearing age uncertain of their status. Meanwhile, silver diamine fluoride-treated lesions can also be covered with GIC or composite. [8]

Not a single adverse event has been reported to the Japanese authorities since they approved silver diamine fluoride (Saforide™, Toyo Seiyaku Kasei Co. Ltd.,

5. STUDIES DONE ON SDF

Studies (authors)
In vivo/in vitro
Results/conclusion.

1.Mei *et al.* [63]
In vitro
The use of 38% SDF inhibited demineralisation and preserved collagen from degradation in demineralised dentin.

2.Mei *et al.* [37]
In vitro
SDF had antimicrobial activity against the cariogenic biofilms and reduced demineralization of dentin.

Mei *et al.* [64]
In vitro
38% SDF inhibits multi-species cariogenic biofilm formation on dentin carious lesions and reduces the demineralization process.

Mei *et al.* [65]
In vitro
SDF application followed by EYL irradiation on a dentin surface increased its resistance to cariogenic biofilm challenge.

Zhang *et al.* [48]
In vivo
Annual application of SDF together with biannual OHE was effective in preventing new root caries and arresting root caries among community-dwelling elderly subjects.

Mathew *et al.* [66]
In vitro
The use of silver diamine fluoride as an endodontic irrigant is feasible as it can effectively remove the microbes present in the canal and circumpulpal dentin.

Actual dose is likely to be much smaller, for example 2.37 mg total for 3 teeth was the largest dose measured in 6 patients. [60] The most frequent application monitored in a clinical trial was weekly for 3 weeks, annually. [62] Thus recommended limit as 1 drop (25 µL) per 10 kg per treatment visit, with weekly intervals at most. [8]

This dose is commensurate with the EPA's allowable short-term exposure of 1.142 mg silver per liter of drinking water for 1-10 days (ATSDR, 1990). Cumulative exposure from lower level acute or chronic silver intake has no real physiologic disease importance, but the bluing of skin in argyria should obviously be avoided. The Environmental Protection Agency set the lifetime exposure conservatively at 1 gram to safely avoid argyria. The highest applied dose for 3 teeth measured in the pharmacokinetic study, 2.37 mg, would enable >400 applications. [60]

The margin of safety for dosing is of paramount concern. Silver and fluoride levels are closely monitored for the U.S. product, and the Health Department of Western Australia conducted a study that found no evidence of fluorosis resulting from long-term proper use of silver diamine fluoride. [8]

Therefore, it is concluded that the development fluorosis after application of the U.S. approved product is not a clinically significant risk.

Osaka, JP) over 80 years ago. The manufacturer estimates that more than 2 million multi-use containers have been sold, including >41,000 units in each of the last three reporting years.[4] In the 9 randomized clinical trials in which silver diamine fluoride was applied to multiple teeth to arrest or prevent dental caries, the only side effect noted was for 3 of 1,493 children or elders monitored for 1-3 years who experienced "a small, mildly painful white lesion in the mucosa, which disappeared at 48 hours without treatment.[20,55,56,43,57,47,48,58,59] The occurrence of reversible localized changes to the oral mucosa was predicted in the first reports of longitudinal studies.[13] No adverse pulpal response was observed.

Gingival responses have been minimal. Gingival contact should be minimized on application. It has been adequate to coat the nearby gingiva with petroleum jelly or cocoa butter. The smallest available microsponge should be used and should be dabbed by the side of the dappen dish to remove excess liquid before application.[8]

In a pharmacokinetic study of silver diamine fluoride application to 3 teeth in each of 6 year olds, no erythema, bleeding, white changes, ulceration, or pigmentation was found after 24 hours. Serum fluoride hardly went up from baseline, while serum silver increased about 10-fold and stayed high past the 4 hours of measurement.[60]

In a 2 site hypersensitivity trial of 126 patients in Peru, at baseline 9% of patients presented redness scores of 2 (1 being normal, 2 being mild to moderate redness, and 3 being severe); and after 1 day 13% in silver diamine fluoride treated patients versus 4% in controls; all redness was gone at 7 days.[61]

Silver allergy is a contraindication. Relative contraindications include any significant desquamative gingivitis or mucositis that disrupts the protective barrier formed by stratified squamous epithelium. Increased absorption and pain would be expected with contact. Heightened caution and use of a protective gingival coating may suffice.[8]

Patients note a transient metallic or bitter taste, however with judicious use the taste and texture response is more favorable than the response to fluoride varnish. Isolating using cotton rolls or application of Vaseline or coca butter is a must.

SDF can stain the skin of the body, clinic surfaces and clothes. The stain caused by SDF on the skin, though not causing any pain, cannot be washed away, and it takes a long time for it to be removed. Spills can be cleaned up immediately with copious water, ethanol, or bleach. [8]

If the skin or clothes have been stained the following procedure is suggested for removing the stain:

(a) Wash out with running water, soap, or high pH solvents such as ammonia water maybe more useful, if immediately after staining.

(b) If the discoloration is not removed and persists, apply the solution of sodium hypochlorite or a bleaching powder (with caution in dyed cloth).

Even a small amount of silver diamine fluoride can cause a "temporary tattoo" to skin (on the patient or provider), like a silver nitrate stain or henna tattoo, and does no harm. Stain on the skin resolves with the natural exfoliation of skin, in 2-14 days. Universal precautions prevent most exposures. Long-term mucosal stain: local argyria akin to an amalgam tattoo has been observed when applying silver nitrate to intra-oral wounds; we anticipate similar stains with submucosal exposure to silver diamine fluoride.

Concerns for fluoride safety are most relevant to chronic exposure, whereas this is an acute exposure. Chronically high systemic fluoride results in dental fluorosis. The ubiquitous use of fluoride-based gas general anaesthetics has shown that the first acute response is transient renal holding, and is rare. Concerns have been raised of poorly controlled silver diamine fluoride concentrations and fluorosis appearing in treated rats. In gaining clearance by the FDA, female and male rat and mouse studies were conducted to determine the lethal dose (LD50) of silver diamine fluoride by oral and subcutaneous administration.

Average LD50 by oral administration was 520 mg/kg, and by subcutaneous administration was 380 mg/kg. The subcutaneous route is taken here as a worst-case scenario. One drop (25 µL) is ample material to treat 5 teeth, and contains 9.5 mg silver diamine fluoride. Assuming the smallest child with caries would be in the range of 10 kg, the dose would be 0.95 mg / kg child. Thus the relative safety margin of using an entire drop on a 10kg child is: 380 mg/kg LD50 / 0.95 mg / kg dose = 400-fold safety margin. [8]

Vasquez *et al.* [60]
In vivo
This preliminary study suggests that serum concentrations of fluoride and silver after topical application of SDF should pose little toxicity risk when used in adults.

Monse *et al.* [58]
In vivo
A one-time application of 38% SDF on the occlusal surfaces of permanent first molars of 6-8 years old children is not an effective method to prevent dentinal caries lesions. ART sealants significantly reduced the onset of caries over a period of 18 months.

Craig *et al.* [15]
In vivo
Product of silver diamine fluoride and potassium iodide has potential as a treatment for dentine hypersensitivity without producing black discolouration.

Zhi *et al.* [55]
In vivo
Arrest of active dentine caries in primary teeth by topical application of SDF solution can be enhanced by increasing the frequency of application from annually to every 6 months, whereas annual paint-on of a flowable glass ionomer can also arrest active dentine caries and may provide a more aesthetic outcome.

Mei *et al.* [67]
In vitro
Greater inhibitory effect on MMPs was found with higher concentration of SDF solution. SDF had more inhibition on MMPs than solutions of NaF and $AgNO_3$ containing equivalent concentration of fluoride respectively.

Quock *et al.* [42]
In vitro
SDF does not adversely affect the bond strength of resin composite to non-carious dentin.

Dos Santos Jr [43]
In vivo

The SDF technique showed better results than IRT with Fuji IX for the arrest of cavities in deciduous teeth, indicating that its use for underprivileged communities may justify a paradigm shift in paediatric dentistry.

Sinha et al. [50]
In vivo

Both glass ionomer (GC Fuji VII) and SDF can be potential indirect pulp capping materials.

Gupta et al. [49]
In vitro

Both SDF and glass ionomer (GC Fuji VII) have remineralizing, re-hardening and antimicrobial efficacy and hence can act as effective IPC materials.

Chu et al. [37]
In vitro

SDF possess an anti-microbial activity against cariogenic biofilm of *S. mutans* or *A. naeslundii* formed on dentin surfaces. SDF slowed down demineralization of dentine. This dual activity could be the reason behind clinical success of SDF.

Hiraishi et al. [68]
In vitro

Both NaOCl and SDF were effective against *E. faecalis* biofilms, with no significant difference. Silver deposits were present on 66.5% of the radicular dentin surfaces after 72-hour application of SDF.

Tan et al. [48]
In vivo

SDF solution proved to be most effective comparing to other solutions ($P<0.001$)

Yee et al. [56]
In vivo

Only the single application of 38% SDF with or without tannic acid was effective in arresting caries after 2 years. 38% was more effective as compared to 12%.

Braga et al. [69]
In vivo

After 3 and 6 months, SDF showed a significantly greater capacity for arresting caries lesions than CTT and GIC. At 18- and 30-month evaluations, no differences were observed among the 3 groups.

Knight et al. [33]
In vitro

SDF/KI treatment of demineralised dentin was more effective in reducing dentin breakdown and the growth of S. mutans as compared to normal dentin. Significantly higher levels of silver and fluoride were deposited within demineralized dentin.

Knight et al. [70]
In vitro

Fluoride uptake was significantly higher in the SDF and KI treated samples compared to the other two samples.

Llodra et al. [57]

In vivo Children in Group 2 developed fewer new caries ($P<0.001$) and more inactive caries at the surface ($P<0.05$) in both the primary teeth and 1st permanent molars.

Chu et al. [14]
In vivo

Children in group 1 developed new caries after 18 months. Group 1 and 2 had about twice the number of caries to be arrested than Group 3,4 and 5 after 30 months ($P<0.001$).

Hihara et al. [71]

In vivo After application of SDF 52% reduction in caries severity and 42% reduction in new caries development.

McDonald and Sheiham [72]
In vivo

No statistically significant difference between groups in caries progression. Caries progressed in only 5% of the SDF/SnF2 group and 11% of the composite resin group.

Suzuki *et al.* [25]

In vitro

SDF showed excellent antibacterial action against cariogenic strains of *S. mutans*

(minimal inhibitory concentration, 0.12 μmole/ml), and completely inhibited the dextran-induced agglutination of *S. mutans* at 0.59 μmole/ml and sucrase activities of *S. mutans* at 0.2 μmole/ml.

Shimizu and Kawagoe [39]

In vivo

No recurrent caries were found when SDF was applied beneath silver amalgam restoration.

Suzuki *et al.* [22]

In vitro

When powdered enamel treated with SDF immersed in saliva CaF_2 gradually decrease while silver thiocyanate retained for longer period.

Penetration of fluoride is about 25μ while silver is 20μ in enamel.

Fluoride uptake was same in all 4 groups but retained fluoride after 1 week was highest for SDF.

Nishino and Massler [41]

In vitro

Application of SDF prior to pit and fissure application lead to decrease the adhesion of Bis-GMA, while did not interfere with polyurethane and cyanoacrylate bonding.

Nishino *et al.* [13]

In vivo

69% lesions in SDF group does not show enlargement as compared to 52% in control. 79% in SDF group shows no increase in pulp ward extension versus 65% in control.

A systematic review was performed to evaluate the efficacy of silver diamine fluoride (SDF) in controlling caries progression in children when compared with active treatments or placebos. A search for randomized clinical trials that evaluated the effectiveness of SDF for caries control in children compared to active treatments or placebos with follow-ups longer than 6 months was performed in PubMed, Scopus, Web of Science, LILACS, BBO, Cochrane Library, and grey literature. [73]

The risk of bias tool from the Cochrane Collaboration was used for quality assessment of the studies. The quality of the evidence was evaluated using the GRADE approach. Meta-analysis was performed on studies considered at low risk of bias. A total of 5,980 articles were identified. Eleven remained in the qualitative synthesis. Five studies were at "low," 2 at "unclear," and 4 studies at "high" risk of bias in the key domains. The studies from which the information could be extracted were included for meta-analysis.

In this way, we collected and systematized data from randomized controlled clinical trials and evaluated the long-term effects of SDF application compared to negative controls or active treatments, focusing on a strict process that evaluates the risk of bias of the available studies and meta-analysing only similar outcomes.

Therefore, in summary the purpose of this systematic review and meta-analysis was to answer the following PICO (participant, intervention, comparator and outcome) question: is SDF more effective than other active treatments/placebo for controlling the progress of active carious lesions in primary teeth and first permanent molars?

The arrestment of caries at 12 months promoted by SDF was 66% higher (95% CI 41–91%; $p < 0.00001$) than by other active material, but it was 154% higher (95% CI 67–85%; $p < 0.00001$) than by placebos.

Overall, the caries arrestment was 89% higher (95% CI 49–138%; $p < 0.00001$) than using active materials/placebo. No heterogeneity was detected. The use of SDF is 89% more effective in controlling/arresting caries than other treatments or placebos. The quality of the evidence was graded as high. [73]

The efficacy of SDF is documented in the literature. Compared to negative control groups like water and saline solution or no treatment at all, SDF is capable of arresting dentin carious lesions in primary teeth. [57]

SDF is more effective than other active treatments or placebo for caries arrestment in primary teeth. The body of evidence was of high quality for primary teeth.

6. AAPD GUIDELINES [74]

* Silver diamine fluoride in this guideline's recommendation refers to 38 percent SDF, the only formula available in the United States.

SETTING

Practitioners must first consider the current standard of care of the setting where SDF therapy is intended for use. Silver diamine fluoride is optimally utilized in the context of a chronic disease management protocol, one that allows for the monitoring of the clinical effectiveness of SDF treatment, disease control, and risk assessment.

PRACTICAL RECOMMENDATION:

Know the setting where SDF is to be used to be consistent with goals of patient-centred care.

INDICATIONS AND USAGE

The following scenarios may be well-suited for the use SDF:
• High caries-risk patients with anterior or posterior active cavitated lesions.
• Cavitated caries lesions in individuals presenting with behavioral or medical management challenges.
• Patients with multiple cavitated caries lesions that may not all be treated in one visit.
• Difficult to treat cavitated dental caries lesions.
• Patients without access to or with difficulty accessing dental care.
• Active cavitated caries lesions with no clinical signs of pulp involvement.

SDF is a valuable caries lesion– arresting tool that can be used in the context of caries management. Evaluate carefully which patients/teeth will benefit from SDF application.

PREPARATION OF PATIENTS AND PRACTITIONERS

Informed consent, particularly highlighting expected staining of treated lesions, potential staining of skin and clothes, and need for reapplication for disease control, is recommended.

The following practices are presented to support patient safety and effectively use SDF:

• Universal precautions.
• No operative intervention (e.g., affected or infected dentin removal) is necessary to achieve caries arrest. [19]
• Protect patient with plastic-lined bib and glasses.
• Cotton roll or other isolation as appropriate.
• Use a plastic dappen dish as SDF corrodes glass and metal.
• Carefully dispose of gloves, cotton rolls, and micro brush into plastic waste bag. Application Carious dentin excavation prior to SDF application is not necessary.

Caries dentin excavation may reduce proportion of arrested caries lesions that become black, and may be considered for esthetic purposes. [20]

Functional indicator of effectiveness (i.e., caries arrest) is when staining on dentinal carious surfaces is visible.

The following steps may vary depending on differing practices, settings, and patients:

• Remove gross debris from cavitation to allow better SDF contact with denatured dentin.
• Minimize contact with gingiva and mucous membranes to avoid potential pigmentation or irritation; consider applying cocoa butter or use cotton rolls to protect surrounding gingival tissues, with care to not inadvertently coat the surfaces of the carious lesion.
• Dry with a gentle flow of compressed air (or use cotton rolls/gauze to dry) affected tooth surfaces.
• Bend micro sponge brush, dip and dab on the side of the dappen dish to remove excess liquid before application; apply SDF directly to only the affected tooth surface.[8]
• Dry with a gentle flow of compressed air for at least one minute.
• Remove excess SDF with gauze, cotton roll, or cotton pellet to minimize systemic absorption. Continue to isolate site for up to three minutes when possible.

PRACTICAL RECOMMENDATION:
No need for surgical intervention (e.g., dentin excavation). SDF application is minimally invasive and easy for the patient and the practitioner. It may be desirable for the caries lesion to be free of gross debris for SDF to have maximum contact with the affected dentin surface.

APPLICATION TIME

An application time of one minute, drying with a gentle flow of compressed air, is recommended. Clinical studies that report application times range from 10 seconds to three minutes. A current review states that application time in clinical studies does not correlate to outcome. More studies are needed to confirm an ideal protocol.

PRACTICAL RECOMMENDATION:
Ideal time of application should be one minute, using a gentle flow of compressed air until liquid is dry. When using shorter application periods, monitor carefully at post-op and re-care to evaluate arrest and consider re-application.

POST-OPERATIVE INSTRUCTIONS

No postoperative limitations are listed by the manufacturer. Eating and drinking immediately following application is acceptable. Patients may brush with fluoridated toothpaste as per regular routine following SDF application. Several SDF clinical trials recommended no eating or drinking for 30 minutes – one hour. [55,56,43]

As patients are used to these recommendations for in-office topical fluoride applications, the recommendation may not be unreasonable to patients, and it may allow for better arrest results. More clinical studies are needed to establish best practices.

APPLICATION FREQUENCY

The effectiveness of one-time SDF application in arresting dental caries lesions ranges from 47 percent to 90 percent, depending on the lesion size and the location of the tooth and the lesion. One study showed that anterior teeth had higher rates of caries lesion arrest than posterior teeth. [75]

The effectiveness of caries lesion arrest, however, decreases over time. After a single application of 38 percent SDF, 50 percent of the arrested surfaces at six months had reverted to active lesions at 24 months. [56] Reapplication may be necessary to sustain arrest. [19,43,55,75]

Annual application of SDF is more effective in arresting caries lesions than application of five percent sodium fluoride varnish four times per year. [20] Increasing frequency of application can increase caries arrest rate. Biannual application of SDF increased the rate of caries lesion arrest compared to annual application. [75]

Studies that had three times per year applications showed higher arrest rates.[57,55,75,76] Frequency of application after baseline has been suggested at three month follow up, and then semi-annual recall visits over two years. One option is to place SDF on active lesions in conjunction with fluoride varnish (FV) on the rest of the dentition, or alternate SDF on caries lesions and FV on the rest of the dentition at three months interval to achieve arrest and prevention in high risk individuals. [77]

Another study recommends one-month post-operative evaluation of treated lesions with optional reapplication as required to achieve arrest of all targeted lesions.[77]

Individuals with high plaque index and lesions with plaque present display lower rates of arrest. Addressing other risk factors like presence of plaque may increase the rate of successful treatment outcomes. [75]

PRACTICAL RECOMMENDATION:

If the setting allows, monitor caries lesion arrest after 2-4-week period and consider reapplication as necessary to achieve arrest of all targeted lesions. Provide re-care monitoring based on patient's disease activity and caries risk level (every three, four, or six months).

Careful monitoring and behavioural intervention to reduce individual risk factors should be part of a comprehensive caries management program that aims not only to sustain arrest of existing caries lesions, but also to prevent new caries lesion development. Adverse reactions No severe pulpal damage or reaction to SDF has been reported.[57,78,79]

However, SDF should not be placed on exposed pulps. Teeth with deep caries lesions should be closely monitored clinically and radiographically.

Serum concentration of fluoride following SDF application per manufacturer recommendations posed little toxicity risk and was below EPA oral reference dose in adults.[60]

The following adverse effects have been noted in the literature:
- Metallic/bitter taste.[8]
- Temporary staining to skin which resolves in 2-14 days.[8]
- Mucosal irritation/lesions resulting from inadvertent contact with SDF, resolved within 48 hours.[57]

ESTHETICS

The hallmark of SDF is a visible dark staining that is a sign of caries arrest on treated dentin lesions. This dark discoloration is permanent unless restored. A recent study that assessed parental perceptions and acceptance of SDF based on the staining found that staining on posterior teeth was more acceptable than on anterior teeth.[80]

Although staining on anterior teeth was perceived as undesirable, most parents preferred this option to avoid the use of advanced behavioural guidance techniques such as sedation or general anaesthesia to deliver traditional restorative care. It was also found that about one-third of parents found SDF treatment unacceptable under any circumstance due to esthetic concerns.

To identify those patients, a thorough informed consent, preferably with photographs that show typical staining, is imperative.[80] Pretreatment of dentin with SDF does not adversely affect bond strength of resin composite to dentin.[81,82]

To improve esthetics, once the disease is controlled and patient's circumstances allow, treated and now-arrested cavitated caries lesions can be restored.[77]

7. CONCLUSION

Silver compounds have been used in dentistry for over a century. Laboratory and clinical studies have shown that they are effective agents particularly to prevent and arrest caries in primary teeth. Efforts to combine silver and fluoride has had greater effects because of its combined mechanism of action. [10]

Silver diamine fluoride is a safe, effective treatment for dental caries across the age spectrum. At UCSF it is indicated for patients with extreme caries risk, patients who cannot undergo a conventional treatment or are too frail to be treated conventionally. It is also useful for patients belonging to despair population with little access to health care. [8]

Since its application does not require dental equipment, it can be used outside the clinical environment. [43] The product is well accepted even by young children since it can be applied without caries removal. [14,19] Therefore, SDF can be considered a user-friendly material for use in dental clinics as well as remote areas, schools or deprived communities. [73]

But there is a unique characteristic that hampers a broader acceptance of this product: the staining of the teeth after SDF application. Therefore, it is important to determine if other non-invasive methods are as effective as SDF in arresting caries in primary teeth and first permanent molars. [73]

If so, these methods could substitute SDF without the disadvantages of teeth staining. The most common treatments that are compared to SDF are fluoride varnish and atraumatic restorative treatment (ART) sealants and restorations

Other than the discoloration and the mild adverse effects which on taking proper precautions can be overcome, modest data compiled from all the literature suggests that can have a significant and substantial benefit in arresting and preventing caries.

By implication, SDF could provide a new quantitative preventive benefit for individuals and populations. Application is simple, the solution is low-cost, and application does not require complex training of the health professionals.

To explore the wider usage of silver compounds, an effort to mask the discolouration should be made.

Thus, SDF appears to meet the criteria of both the WHO Millennium Goals, and the Institute of Medicine's criteria for 21st century medicine (Institute of Medicine, 2001). However, broader study sets are required to investigate alternative protocols and newer horizons of research for its use as other delivery systems, for occlusal, proximal, and root caries.

As well, the applications of SDF for treating tooth sensitivity, periodontal pockets and pulpal infections need to be evaluated by further research. [9]

8. BIBLIOGRAPHY

1. Chu CH, Fung DS, Lo EC. Dental public health: dental caries status of preschool children in Hong Kong. British dental journal. 1999 Dec;187(11):616.

2. Shah S, Bhaskar V, Venkatraghavan K, Choudhary P, Trivedi K. Silver diamine fluoride: a review and current applications. Journal of Advanced Oral Research. 2014 Jan;5(1):25-35.

3. Bedi R, Sardo-Infirri J. Oral health care in disadvantaged communities. London: FDI World,1999.

4. Hiiri A, Ahovuo-Saloranta A, Nordblad A, Mäkelä M. Pit and fissure sealants versus fluoride varnishes for preventing dental decay in children and adolescents. Cochrane Database of Systematic Reviews. 2010(3)

5. Featherstone JD. Prevention and reversal of dental caries: role of low level fluoride. Community dentistry and oral epidemiology. 1999 Feb;27(1):31-40.

6. Hamilton IR. Biochemical effects of fluoride on oral bacteria. Journal of dental research. 1990 Feb;69(2_suppl):660-7.

7. Cate JM. Current concepts on the theories of the mechanism of action of fluoride. Acta Odontologica Scandinavica. 1999 Jan 1;57(6):325-9.

8. Horst JA, Ellenikiotis H, Milgrom PM, UCSF Silver Caries Arrest Committee. UCSF protocol for caries arrest using silver diamine fluoride: rationale, indications, and consent. Journal of the California Dental Association. 2016 Jan;44(1):16.

9. Rosenblatt A, Stamford TC, Niederman R. Silver diamine fluoride: a caries "silver-fluoride bullet". Journal of dental research. 2009 Feb;88(2):116-25.

10. Peng JY, Botelho MG, Matinlinna JP. Silver compounds used in dentistry for caries management: a review. Journal of dentistry. 2012 Jul 1;40(7):531-41.

11. Klasen HJ. A historical review of the use of silver in the treatment of burns. II. Renewed interest for silver. Burns. 2000 Mar 1;26(2):131-8.

12. Moyer CA, BRENTANO L, GRAVENS DL, MARGRAF HW, MONAFO . Treatment of large human burns with 0.5% silver nitrate solution. Archives of surgery. 1965 Jun 1;90(6):812-67.

13. Yamaga R. Diamine silver fluoride and its clinical application. J Osaka Univ Dent Sch. 1972; 12:1-20.

14. Chu CH, Lo EC. Promoting caries arrest in children with silver diamine fluoride: a review. Oral health & preventive dentistry. 2008 Sep 1;6(4):315-321

15. Craig GG, Knight GM, McIntyre JM. Clinical evaluation of diamine silver fluoride/potassium iodide as a dentine desensitizing agent. A pilot study. Australian dental journal. 2012 Sep;57(3):308-11.

16. Klein U, Kanellis MJ, Drake D. Effects of four anticaries agents on lesion depth progression in an in vitro caries model. Pediatr Dent. 1999 May;21(3):176-80.

17. Craig GG, Powell KR, Cooper MH. Caries progression in primary molars: 24-month results from a minimal treatment programme. Community dentistry and oral epidemiology. 1981 Dec;9(6):260-5.

18. Green E. A clinical evaluation of two methods of caries prevention in newly-erupted first permanent molars. Australian dental journal. 1989 Oct;34(5):407-9.

19. Chu CH, Lo EC, Lin HC. Effectiveness of silver diamine fluoride and sodium fluoride varnish in arresting dentin caries in Chinese pre-school children. Journal of dental research. 2002 Nov;81(11):767-70.

20. Lo EC, Chu CH, Lin HC. A community-based caries control program for pre-school children using topical fluorides: 18-month results. Journal of dental research. 2001 Dec;80(12):2071-4.

21. Selvig KA. Ultrastructural changes in human dentine exposed to a weak acid. Archives of oral biology. 1968 Jul 1;13(7):719-IN9.

22. Suzuki T. Effects of diammine silver fluoride on tooth enamel. J Osaka Univ Dent Sch. 1974; 14:61-72.

23. Kani T. X-ray diffraction studies on effect of fluoride on restoration of lattice imperfections of apatite crystals. [Osaka Daigaku shigaku zasshi] The journal of Osaka University Dental Society. 1970 Jun;15(1):42-56

24. Okazaki M, Takahashi J, Kumura H. Crystal growth of fluoridated hydroxyapatites inhibited in the presence of gelatin. The Journal of Osaka University Dental School. 1989 Dec; 29:47-52.

25. Suzuki T, Sobue S, Suginaka H. Mechanism of antiplaque action of diamine silver fluoride. J Osaka Univ Dent Sch. 1976; 16:87-95.

26. Sunada I, Kuriyama S, Komamura T. Resistance to acid and enzyme of dentin treated by metal ion ionophoresis. Jap. J. Conserv. Dent. 1962; 5:6-10.

27. Yanagida I, Nishino M, Hano T. Effects of diammine silver fluoride on organic components of dentin of deciduous teeth. Jap. J. Pedo. 1971; 9:39-46.

28. Lansdown AB. Silver I: its antibacterial properties and mechanism of action. Journal of wound care. 2002 Apr;11(4):125-30.

29. Wu MY, Suryanarayanan K, Van Ooij WJ, Oerther DB. Using microbial genomics to evaluate the effectiveness of silver to prevent biofilm formation. Water science and technology. 2007 Apr 1;55(8-9):413-9.

30. Oppermann RV, Rölla G. Effect of some polyvalent cations on the acidogenicity of dental plaque in vivo. Caries research. 1980;14(6):422-7.

31. Lansdown AB. Silver in health care: antimicrobial effects and safety in use. In Biofunctional textiles and the skin 2006 (Vol. 33, pp. 17-34). Karger Publishers.

32. Knight GM, McIntyre JM, Craig GG, Zilm PS, Gully NJ. Inability to form a biofilm of Streptococcus mutans on silver fluoride-and potassium iodide-treated demineralized dentin. Quintessence International. 2009 Feb 1;40(2).

33. Knight GM, McIntyre JM, Craig GG, Zilm PS, Gully NJ. An in vitro model to measure the effect of a silver fluoride and potassium iodide treatment on the permeability of demineralized dentine to Streptococcus mutans. Australian dental journal. 2005 Dec;50(4):242-5.

34. Knight GM, McIntyre JM, Craig GG, Mulyani, Zilm PS, Gully NJ. Differences between normal and demineralized dentine pretreated with silver fluoride and potassium iodide after an in vitro challenge by Streptococcus mutans. Australian dental journal. 2007 Mar;52(1):16-21.

35. Wakshlak RB, Pedahzur R, Avnir D. Antibacterial activity of silver-killed bacteria: the" zombies" effect. Scientific reports. 2015 Apr 23; 5:9555.

36. Mohammadi N, Far MH. Effect of fluoridated varnish and silver diamine fluoride on enamel demineralization resistance in primary dentition. Journal of Indian Society of Pedodontics and Preventive Dentistry. 2018 Jul 1;36(3):257.

37. Chu CH, Mei LE, Seneviratne CJ, Lo EC. Effects of silver diamine fluoride on dentine carious lesions induced by Streptococcus mutans and Actinomyces naeslundii biofilms. International journal of paediatric dentistry. 2012 Jan;22(1):2-10.

38. Anusavice KJ, Shen C, Rawls HR, editors. Phillips' science of dental materials. Elsevier Health Sciences; 2012 Sep 27.

39. Shimizu A. A clinical study of effect of diamine silver fluoride on recurrent caries. J Osaka Univ Dent Sch. 1976; 16:103-9.

40. Sato R, Sailo Y. Clinical application of silver ammonia fluoride (SAFORIDE) to children. The Nippon Dental Review1970. 1970; 332:66-7.

41. Nishino M, Massler M. Immunization of caries-susceptible pits and fissures with a diammine silver fluoride solution. The Journal of pedodontics. 1977;2(1):16.

42. Quock RL, Patel SA, Falcao FA, Barros JA. Is a drill-less dental filling possible? Medical hypotheses. 2011 Sep 1;77(3):315-7.

43. dos Santos Jr VE, De Vasconcelos FM, Ribeiro AG, Rosenblatt A. Paradigm shift in the effective treatment of caries in schoolchildren at risk. International dental journal. 2012 Feb;62(1):47-51.

44. Griffin SO, Griffin PM, Swann JL, Zlobin N. Estimating rates of new root caries in older adults. Journal of dental research. 2004 Aug;83(8):634-8.

45. Chalmers JM, Hodge C, Fuss JM, Spencer AJ, Carter KD. The prevalence and experience of oral diseases in Adelaide nursing home residents. Australian dental journal. 2002 Jun;47(2):123-30.

46. Lo EC, Luo Y, Dyson JE. Oral health status of institutionalised elderly in Hong Kong. Community dental health. 2004 Sep;21(3):224-6.

47. Tan HP, Lo EC, Dyson JE, Luo Y, Corbet EF. A randomized trial on root caries prevention in elders. Journal of dental research. 2010 Oct;89(10):1086-90.

48. Zhang W, McGrath C, Lo EC, Li JY. Silver diamine fluoride and education to prevent and arrest root caries among community-dwelling elders. Caries research. 2013;47(4):284-90.

49. Gupta A, Sinha N, Logani A, Shah N. An ex vivo study to evaluate the remineralizing and antimicrobial efficacy of silver diamine fluoride and glass ionomer cement type VII for their proposed use as indirect pulp capping materials–Part I. Journal of conservative dentistry: JCD. 2011 Apr;14(2):113.

50. Sinha N, Gupta A, Logani A, Shah N. Remineralizing efficacy of silver diamine fluoride and glass ionomer type VII for their proposed use as indirect pulp

capping materials–Part II (A clinical study). Journal of conservative dentistry: JCD. 2011 Jul;14(3):233.

51. Duangthip D, Gao SS, Chen KJ, Lo EC, Chu CH. Oral health-related quality of life of preschool children receiving silver diamine fluoride therapy: A prospective 6-month study. Journal of dentistry. 2019 Feb 1; 81:27-32.

52. Magno MB, Silva LP, Ferreira DM, Barja-Fidalgo F, Fonseca-Gonçalves A. Aesthetic perception, acceptability and satisfaction in the treatment of caries lesions with silver diamine fluoride: A scoping review. International journal of paediatric dentistry. 2019 May;29(3):257-66.

53. Li R, Lo EC, Chu CH, Liu B. Preventing and arresting root caries through silver diammine fluoride applications. Journal of Dental Research. 2014.

54. Mei ML, Lo EC, Chu CH. Clinical use of silver diamine fluoride in dental treatment. Compend Contin Educ Dent. 2016 Feb;37(2):93-8.

55. Zhi QH, Lo EC, Lin HC. Randomized clinical trial on effectiveness of silver diamine fluoride and glass ionomer in arresting dentine caries in preschool children. Journal of dentistry. 2012 Nov 1;40(11):962-7.

56. Yee R, Holmgren C, Mulder J, Lama D, Walker D, van Palenstein Helderman W. Efficacy of silver diamine fluoride for arresting caries treatment. Journal of dental research. 2009 Jul;88(7):644-7.

57. Llodra JC, Rodriguez A, Ferrer B, Menardia V, Ramos T, Morato M. Efficacy of silver diamine fluoride for caries reduction in primary teeth and first permanent molars of schoolchildren: 36-month clinical trial. Journal of dental research. 2005 Aug;84(8):721-4.

58. Monse B, Heinrich-Weltzien R, Mulder J, Holmgren C, van Palenstein Helderman WH. Caries preventive efficacy of silver diammine fluoride (SDF) and ART sealants in a school-based daily fluoride tooth brushing program in the Philippines. BMC oral health. 2012 Dec;12(1):52.

59. Ma RL. Clinical observation of treatment of tooth hypersensitivity with silver ammonia fluoride solution.Chinese journal of stomatology. 1993 Jan;28(1):30.

60. Vasquez E, Zegarra G, Chirinos E, Castillo JL, Taves DR, Watson GE, Dills R, Mancl LL, Milgrom P. Short term serum pharmacokinetics of diammine silver fluoride after oral application. BMC Oral Health. 2012 Dec;12(1):60.

61. Castillo JL, Rivera S, Aparicio T, Lazo R, Aw TC, Mancl LL, Milgrom P. The short-term effects of diammine silver fluoride on tooth sensitivity: a randomized controlled trial. Journal of dental research. 2011 Feb;90(2):203-8.

62. Duangthip D, Fung MH, Wong MC, Chu CH, Lo EC. Adverse effects of silver diamine fluoride treatment among preschool children. Journal of dental research. 2018 Apr;97(4):395-401.

63. Mei ML, Ito L, Cao Y, Li QL, Lo EC, Chu CH. Inhibitory effect of silver diamine fluoride on dentine demineralisation and collagen degradation. Journal of dentistry. 2013 Sep 1;41(9):809-17.

64. Mei ML, Li QL, Chu CH, Lo EM, Samaranayake LP. Antibacterial effects of silver diamine fluoride on multi-species cariogenic biofilm on caries. Annals of clinical microbiology and antimicrobials. 2013 Jan;12(1):4.

65. Mei ML, Ito L, Chu CH, Lo EC, Zhang CF. Prevention of dentine caries using silver diamine fluoride application followed by Er: YAG laser irradiation: an in vitro study. Lasers in medical science. 2014 Nov 1;29(6):1785-91.

66. Mathew VB, Madhusudhana K, Sivakumar N, Venugopal T, Reddy RK. Anti-microbial efficiency of silver diamine fluoride as an endodontic medicament–An ex vivo study. Contemporary clinical dentistry. 2012 Jul;3(3):262.

67. Mei ML, Ito L, Cao Y, Li QL, Chu CH, Lo EC. The inhibitory effects of silver diamine fluorides on cysteine cathepsins. Journal of dentistry. 2014 Mar 1;42(3):329-35.

68. Hiraishi N, Yiu CK, King NM, Tagami J, Tay FR. Antimicrobial efficacy of 3.8% silver diamine fluoride and its effect on root dentin. Journal of endodontics. 2010 Jun 1;36(6):1026-9.

69. Braga MM, Mendes FM, De Benedetto MS, Imparato JC. Effect of silver diammine fluoride on incipient caries lesions in erupting permanent first molars: a pilot study. Journal of Dentistry for Children. 2009 Mar 15;76(1):28-33.

70. Knight GM, Mclntyre JM, Craig GG, Mulyani. Ion uptake into demineralized dentine from glass ionomer cement following pretreatment with silver fluoride and potassium iodide. Australian dental journal. 2006 Sep;51(3):237-41.

71. Hihara T, Nishino M, Yasutomi Y, Tominaga T, Mori Y, Arita K. Effects of diammine silver fluoride on arrestment and prevention of caries in primary tooth. Dentistry in Japan. 1994 Dec; 31:93-5.

72. McDonald SP, Sheiham A. A clinical comparison of non-traumatic methods of treating dental caries. International dental journal. 1994 Oct;44(5):465-70.

73. Chibinski AC, Wambier LM, Feltrin J, Loguercio AD, Wambier DS, Reis A. Silver diamine fluoride has efficacy in controlling caries progression in primary teeth: a systematic review and meta-analysis. Caries research. 2017;51(5):527-41.

74. Crystal YO, Niederman R. Silver diamine fluoride treatment considerations in children's caries management. Pediatric dentistry. 2016 Nov 15;38(7):466-71.

75. Fung MH, Duangthip D, Wong MC, Lo EC, Chu CH. Arresting dentine caries with different concentration and periodicity of silver diamine fluoride. JDR Clinical & Translational Research. 2016 Jul;1(2):143-52.

76. Duangthip D, Chu CH, Lo EC. A randomized clinical trial on arresting dentine caries in preschool children by topical fluorides—18 month results. Journal of dentistry. 2016 Jan 1; 44:57-63.

77. Crystal YO, Marghalani AA, Ureles SD, Wright JT, Sulyanto R, Divaris K, Fontana M, Graham L. Use of silver diamine fluoride for dental caries management in children and adolescents, including those with special health care needs. Pediatric dentistry. 2017 Sep 15;39(5):135E-45E.

78. Nishino M. Effect of topically applied ammoniacal silver fluoride on dental caries in children. J Osaka Univ Dent Sch. 1969; 9:149-55.

79. Okuyama T. On the penetration of diammine silver fluoride into the carious dentin of deciduous teeth (author's transl). Shigaku= Odontology; journal of Nihon Dental College. 1974 Feb;61(6):1048.

80. Crystal YO, Janal MN, Hamilton DS, Niederman R. Parental perceptions and acceptance of silver diamine fluoride staining. The Journal of the American Dental Association. 2017 Jul 1;148(7):510-8.

81. Quock RL, Barros JA, Yang SW, Patel SA. Effect of silver diamine fluoride on microtensile bond strength to dentin. Operative dentistry. 2012 Oct;37(6):610-6.

82. Selvaraj K, Sampath V, Sujatha V, Mahalaxmi S. Evaluation of microshear bond strength and nanoleakage of etch-and-rinse and self-etch adhesives to dentin pretreated with silver diamine fluoride/potassium iodide: An in vitro study. Indian Journal of Dental Research. 2016 Jul 1;27(4):421.

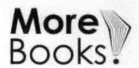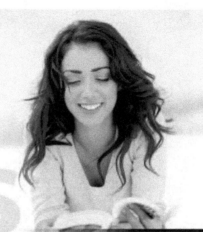

I want morebooks!

Buy your books fast and straightforward online - at one of world's fastest growing online book stores! Environmentally sound due to Print-on-Demand technologies.

Buy your books online at
www.morebooks.shop

Kaufen Sie Ihre Bücher schnell und unkompliziert online – auf einer der am schnellsten wachsenden Buchhandelsplattformen weltweit! Dank Print-On-Demand umwelt- und ressourcenschonend produziert.

Bücher schneller online kaufen
www.morebooks.shop

KS OmniScriptum Publishing
Brivibas gatve 197
LV-1039 Riga, Latvia
Telefax: +371 686 204 55

info@omniscriptum.com
www.omniscriptum.com

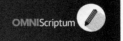

Printed in the USA
CPSIA information can be obtained
at www.ICGtesting.com
LVHW09020505092 3
757239LV00007B/236